Reset with Intermittent Fasting

A 12-Week Workbook and Journal to Help You Lose Weight, Regain Energy, and Take Back Your Health for Longevity

AF777649

Ellen Sedge

RESET

Impisi™ Media

Reset with Intermittent Fasting: A 12-Week Workbook and Journal to Help You Lose Weight, Regain Energy, and Take Back Your Health for Longevity

Copyright © 2025 by Impisi™ Media

All rights reserved. No part of this publication may be reproduced, distributed, or transmitted in any form or by any means, including photocopying, recording, or other electronic or mechanical methods, without the prior written permission of the publisher, except in the case of brief quotations embodied in critical reviews and certain other noncommercial uses permitted by copyright law.

ISBN: 978-1-965722-17-6 (Paperback)
ISBN: 978-1-965722-18-3 (Hardcover)
ISBN: 978-1-965722-19-0 (Spiral)

Book design by Impisi™ Media

First printing edition 2025.

Published by Impisi™ Media LLC in the United States of America.
5830 E 2ND ST, STE 7000, CASPER, WY 82609 +1 (307) 275 8745

www.impisimedia.com

Impisi™ is subject to a trademark application by Impisi Media LLC.

ALSO BY THE PUBLISHER

SMALL BUSINESS SERIES

Should You Start a Business or Not?

Business Entry: Starting vs Buying

3 Keys to Maximize Profitability

SMART WORK-LIFE SERIES

Mastering Time for Productivity

The Wolf's Edge - Strategies for Intelligent Living

Reset with Intermittent Fasting

SCAN ME

Scan the QR code to to join our newsletter and receive updates on new releases and book resources.

To the ones embracing
change, trusting the
process, and showing
up for themselves
every day.

TABLE OF CONTENTS

Dear Journeyer,

First, let me congratulate you on making this decision. By choosing to embrace intermittent fasting (IF), you are not just changing when you eat, you are embarking on a profound journey of self-discovery, healing, and transformation. Intermittent fasting is more than a tool for weight loss; it is a powerful shift in how you care for your body, mind, and spirit.

This journey will reveal clarity, resilience, and inner strength you may not have fully recognized before. There will be days when fasting feels effortless, and others when challenges arise. Let those moments be opportunities for growth, patience, and self-compassion. Every step you take brings you closer to a healthier, more balanced version of yourself.

This journal was designed with you in mind, not as a rigid set of tick boxes, but as a space for reflection, awareness, and personal wisdom. Here, you can capture your thoughts, emotions, victories, and lessons. As you progress, you may find that the words you write reveal insights about yourself that go beyond fasting. They may reflect renewed confidence, emotional healing, and deeper self-trust.

I am truly cheering you on. Trust the process. Your body knows what to do, and so do you. This is your journey, embrace it fully, with courage and grace.

You've got this.
With love,

Ellen

HOW TO USE THIS JOURNAL

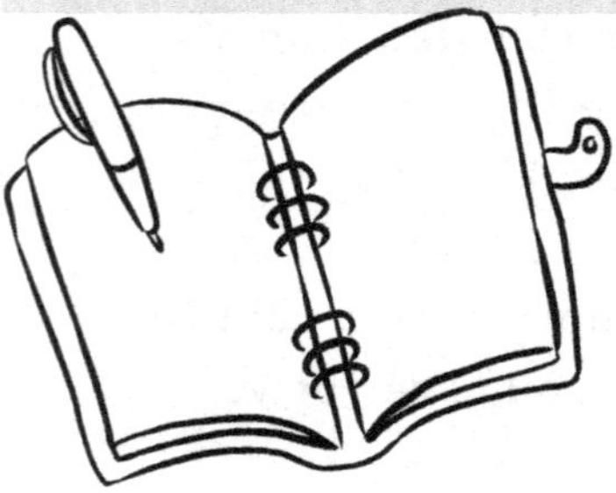

This journal was created to support your journey with intermittent fasting, whether you are taking your very first steps or refining an already established routine.

Unlike typical journals filled with tick boxes, emojis, or overly prescriptive prompts, this one follows a user respecting design. It offers you the freedom to capture your experience in a way that feels natural and personal.

Each of the twelve weeks includes ten thoughtfully structured pages. You will find a journaling page for every day, from Monday to Sunday. These pages include broad headings such as “What went well today” or “Describe your emotions during the fast,” inviting you to record whatever is meaningful to you.

That might include your fasting window, meals, mood, sleep, energy levels, or a simple note about how your day went. There is no right or wrong way to use these pages.

In addition to the daily pages, each week includes three supporting pages. “The Week That Was” provides an opportunity to reflect on your experiences and emotional journey. “Planning the Week Ahead” enables you to set gentle intentions, note your goals, or mentally prepare for any upcoming changes.

A motivational quote page offers inspiration to carry you through the week with a fresh perspective.

This is more than a logbook. It is a place to notice patterns, connect with your inner wisdom, and record both the challenges and the victories along the way. It is designed to work with you, not against you, and to hold space for whatever your path may bring.

To further support your practice, this journal offers something truly unique; a workbook-style experience paired with full access to the Intermittent Fasting Hub (IF HUB), an exclusive online resource for journal owners. The IF HUB is equivalent in depth to a complete book on fasting, thoughtfully structured into easy-to-follow topics.

Each guide can be read online, this means all the information you need is available at your fingertips, so your journal can remain clean, open, and centered on your unique experience.

Both the journal and IF HUB were inspired by a real-life couple who embraced intermittent fasting as part of a lasting lifestyle change. Their experience, reflections, and insights helped shape every element you'll find here. What you hold in your hands is not theory, it's the result of lived commitment.

Let this journal become your companion.
Use it daily, use it gently, and above all,
use it in a way that honors your journey.

HOW TO ACCESS AND USE THE IF HUB

Now that you're familiar with how to use your journal, it's time to unlock even more support and inspiration designed to help you succeed.

The IF HUB is your personal online companion, exclusively created for journal owners like you. The Hub is packed with in-depth information in the form of articles which can be read online from any device for your convenience.

There is also a handy FAQ section that answers many of the questions you might have along the way.

While your journal gives you a strong foundation for tracking your intermittent fasting journey, the IF HUB takes things a step further by providing detailed guidance and additional resources to deepen your understanding and keep you motivated every step of the way.

By registering your account, you gain access to this rich collection of resources, giving you all the tools and answers you need right at your fingertips.

This way, your journal pages can stay clean, open, and focused on your unique experience, while the IF HUB fills in the details and supports you in ways a journal alone can't.

Together, they create a complete system designed to guide you toward your goals with confidence and clarity.

ALREADY HAVE AN ACCOUNT?

If you've already registered an account on impisimedia.com, getting into the IF HUB is super easy:

- Login to your account, you'll land on your MY ACCOUNT page
- Look for the Access Codes menu on the left-hand side and click it.
- You'll see a field labeled IF Hub, enter your special access code from this journal there.
- Click SUBMIT CODE and voilà! You'll be granted access to all the awesome IF HUB content.

! Access code on page 13

NEW USER REGISTRATION

If this is your first time, no worries! Here's how to get started:

- Head to https://impisimedia.com and click MY ACCOUNT from the menu.
- Click REGISTER on the dropdown menu.
- Fill out the registration form and be sure to enter the access code from this journal in the designated field.
- Submit the form and check your email inbox for a verification message. (Make sure to also check your spam folder)
- Click the link in that email to confirm your account. Once verified, your account will be created and you'll get full access to the IF HUB.

IF HUB CONTENT LAYOUT

1

OUR JOURNEY

Explore our personal journey with Intermittent Fasting and how it transformed our health. Learn how to use our specially designed IF Journal to track your progress and stay motivated throughout your fasting experience.

2

BEGINNERS GUIDE TO IF

Learn the basics of intermittent fasting, how it compares to traditional diets, its key health benefits, and find recommended resources to help you get started on your fasting journey.

3

FASTING PLANS & METHODS

Discover different fasting plans, how to choose the right one for your lifestyle, and access a handy Excel fasting planner to track your progress and stay on track with your goals.

4

FOOD & EATING GUIDELINES

Learn which foods support or hinder fasting, uncover hidden sugars, explore different diets, and understand how coffee affects autophagy. Get tips on breaking your fast and optimizing fat-burning nutrition.

Access Code:
RLIFE

5

SMART MEAL PLANNING

Create an effective meal plan with ready-to-use templates for OMAD and two-meal fasting. Use our easy meal planning blueprint document to simplify your meals and stay on track with your fasting goals.

6

TRACK YOUR PROGRESS

Stay on top of your fasting journey with progress tracking tools, weight loss targets, and helpful apps. Download an Excel tracker and explore useful products to support your goals.

7

LIVING WITH INTENTION: A MINDFUL APPROACH

Intermittent Fasting is more than a diet, it's a mindset. Explore how aligning body, mind, and soul through gratitude and awareness creates lasting change and a deeper sense of well-being.

8

EXCLUSIVE OFFER TO MEMBERS

If you order your next journal from the Impisi Media website, you will receive a 15% discount by using the code website15 at checkout.

9 FREQUENTLY ASKED QUESTIONS (FAQs)

SUMMARY OF FOODS TO EMBRACE DURING FASTING

PROTEIN SOURCES

- Meats (chicken, turkey, beef, pork)
- Fatty fish (salmon, mackerel, sardines)
- Eggs, nuts & seeds in moderation

CARBS & FIBER

- Non-starchy vegetables (broccoli, kale, spinach)
- Berries (strawberries, raspberries, blackberries)
- Legumes (lentils, beans, all in moderation)

NUTRIENTS & MINERALS

- Leafy greens (spinach, Swiss chard, Brussels sprouts)
- Healthy fats (avocados, avocado oil, olive oil, coconut oil)
- Fermented foods (unsweetened yogurt, sauerkraut, kimchi)

SUMMARY OF FOODS TO AVOID DURING FASTING

PROTEIN SOURCES

- Processed meats (sausages, hot dogs, deli meats)
- Breaded or fried proteins

CARBS & FIBER

- Refined grains (white bread, pasta, rice)
- Sugary foods (desserts, candy, sodas)
- Starchy vegetables (potatoes, corn, peas)

NUTRIENTS & MINERALS

- Highly processed foods (chips, packaged snacks)
- Sugary sauces (ketchup, BBQ sauce, dressings)

SUMMARY OF FAT BURNING FOOD GROUPS

MEAT, FISH & POULTRY

Rich in high-quality protein, these foods support muscle maintenance and boost metabolism through the thermic effect of food.

EGGS & AVOCADO

Eggs offer complete protein and healthy fats, while avocados are loaded with fiber and monounsaturated fats that promote satiety and stable energy.

HEALTHY FATS

Sources like extra virgin olive oil, coconut oil, avocado oil and MCT oil help reduce cravings, support hormone function, and encourage fat-burning through steady energy release.

NON-STARCHY VEGETABLES

Leafy greens like lettuce, kale, spinach, and Swiss chard. Non-leafy vegetables such as broccoli, cauliflower, Brussels sprouts, cabbage, and bell peppers.

FUNCTIONAL FOODS

Items like bone broth, dark chocolate and apple cider vinegar support metabolism, reduce inflammation, and improve gut health.

FERMENTED FOODS

Dairy based fermented foods include sour cream, plain and unflavored kefir, and yogurt. Vegetable fermented foods like sauerkraut and kimchi.

NUTS & SEEDS

Almonds, macadamias, walnuts, and pecans. Seeds such as flaxseeds, chia seeds, pumpkin seeds, and hemp seeds.

SUMMARY OF RECOMMENDED FOODS TO BREAK A FAST

BONE BROTH

A small serving of bone broth is excellent for rehydration and providing electrolytes, collagen, and amino acids to ease digestion.

COOKED VEGETABLES

Lightly steamed or roasted vegetables like zucchini, spinach, or asparagus are easy to digest and provide fiber, vitamins, and minerals.

FERMENTED FOODS

Options like plain Greek yogurt, kefir, or a small serving of sauerkraut or kimchi support gut health by introducing probiotics.

AVOCADO

Rich in healthy fats and fiber, avocado is a satisfying option that's easy on the stomach and helps maintain satiety.

LEAN PROTEIN

Small portions of chicken or fish provide protein without overwhelming the digestive system. Eggs, boiled or scrambled, are also excellent choices.

HEALTHY FATS

Incorporate fats like extra virgin olive oil, coconut oil, avocado oil, or a small handful of nuts to promote satiety and energy without spiking blood sugar.

SUMMARY OF FOODS TO AVOID WHEN BREAKING A FAST

HIGH-SUGAR FOODS

Even natural options like fruits with a high glycemic index (e.g., bananas or mangoes) should be consumed later, after the digestive system has adjusted.

FRIED OR GREASY FOODS

These can be difficult to digest and lead to bloating or discomfort.

LARGE PORTIONS

Overeating immediately after fasting can strain your digestive system and lead to fatigue.

CARBONATED DRINKS

Sodas or sparkling water can cause bloating, especially on an empty stomach.

HOW TO HANDLE OMAD

1. **Start Light**: Begin with a small portion of bone broth or plain Greek yoghurt, a boiled egg, or a handful of nuts to prepare your stomach for digestion.
2. **Incorporate Protein and Fats**: Follow up with a main course that includes protein paired with healthy fats (e.g., avocado or olive oil) and a generous portion of non- starchy vegetables. This combination ensures satiety and provides sustained energy.
3. **Stay Hydrated**: Drink plenty of water before and during your meal to avoid overeating. Adding a pinch of salt to your water can help replenish electrolytes.
4. **Space It Out**: If possible, spread your meal over 2–4 hours instead of eating everything in one sitting. This helps ease digestion and prevents discomfort.

SUMMARY OF FASTING PLANS AND TYPES

THE 16/8 PLAN

It involves fasting for 16 hours and eating within an 8-hour window. For example, if you stop eating at 8:00 PM, your next meal wouldn't be until 12:00 PM the following day.

THE 18/6 PLAN

The 18/6 plan extends the fasting window by two hours and narrows the eating window to six hours.

THE 20/4 PLAN

The 20/4 plan, often called the Warrior Diet, involves fasting for 20 hours and eating within a 4-hour window.

THE OMAD PLAN (ONE MEAL A DAY)

With an 8:00 PM starting point, you would fast for 22–23 hours, breaking the fast with a single meal around 6:00–7:00 PM the next day. OMAD simplifies the eating process by creating this extended fasting window, which provides profound benefits like enhanced fat-burning and deeper autophagy.

THE ALTERNATE-DAY METHOD

Alternate-day fasting involves fasting every other day. On fasting days, some people choose to consume minimal calories (around 500), while others abstain from eating entirely.

THE EAT-STOP-EAT METHOD

Eat-Stop-Eat is an intermittent fasting method where you fast for 24 hours once or twice a week.

MANAGING YOUR HUNGER

Hunger is often misunderstood. It's not an emergency; it's a temporary sensation, a wave that rises and falls. In modern life, we've been conditioned to think we need to eat at the first sign of hunger, but fasting teaches us something different: hunger is fluid and it passes.

During a fast, hunger is usually strongest at the times you'd typically eat. This is habit-driven hunger, not an actual physical need. After a while, your body adapts, and hunger fades. Drinking water, black coffee, or herbal tea can help, as can staying engaged in an activity; sometimes, hunger is simply boredom in disguise.

If you experience persistent hunger, it could be due to electrolyte imbalances. A pinch of salt in a glass of water or a teaspoon of pure lemon or lime juice in your water bottle can often settle things.

If you truly need something to tie you over, a teaspoon of butter, extra virgin olive oil, or avocado oil stirred into black coffee provides satiety with minimal impact on fasting benefits.

Overcoming hunger isn't about fighting it; it's about understanding it. The more you fast, the more you'll recognize that hunger is not a constant but a passing signal. Trust that your body knows what to do, and let the waves of hunger come and go.

You are in control.

! Remember to use your weight tracker.
Download your Excel file from the hub.

"The best investment you will ever make is in yourself."

This journey isn't just about fasting; it's about building confidence, resilience, and a life that feels good to live.

Keep going.

LOOK AT ME!

Paste your picture here

Before

Weight _______________

BMI __________________

Body fat ______________

Chest _________________

Waist _________________

Hips __________________

Thighs ________________

Paste your picture here

After

Weight _______________

BMI __________________

Body fat ______________

Chest _________________

Waist _________________

Hips __________________

Thighs ________________

DAILY AFFIRMATIONS FOR SUCCESS

Introduction

Your mindset shapes your journey. Use affirmations every day to stay motivated, embrace consistency, and celebrate progress, one fast at a time.

About Affirmations

Affirmations are powerful, positive statements that help reinforce a strong mindset, boost confidence, and keep you focused on your goals. They serve as reminders of your intentions, strengths, and abilities, especially on days when motivation feels low.

To get the most out of affirmations:

✓ Use them daily: Repeating affirmations consistently strengthens your mindset and commitment.

✓ Say them out loud in front of a mirror: Looking yourself in the eye while affirming your goals builds confidence and reinforces belief.

✓ Visualize them as true: Picture yourself achieving what you affirm—see the progress, feel the success.

✓ Write them down: Keeping small affirmation cards or sticky notes in visible places (mirror, desk, fridge) helps reinforce them throughout the day.

✓ Believe in them: Even if it feels unnatural at first, trust that your mindset shapes your reality.

Affirmations are not just words, they are intentions turned into action. Use them to strengthen your commitment to your fasting journey, your health, and your personal growth.

Affirmation Suggestions

- I am in control of my body and my choices.
- Every fast I complete makes me stronger and healthier.
- Hunger is temporary; my goals are permanent.
- I trust my body to adapt and thrive.
- Each day, I am becoming the best version of myself.
- I fuel my body with nourishing foods and mindful habits.
- I am patient with my progress because I know it's worth it.
- I respect my body and give it the care it deserves.
- I choose consistency over perfection.
- I am creating a lifestyle that supports my well-being.
- My health is improving with every mindful decision.
- I embrace challenges as opportunities to grow.
- I listen to my body and honor what it needs.
- I am capable, disciplined, and committed to my journey.
- Success is built one small, consistent step at a time.

Final Thoughts

Choose three affirmations that resonate with you the most and repeat them daily. Just like fasting, consistency matters more than perfection; focus on the mindset that will support your journey, and the results will follow.

LIVING WITH INTENTION: A MINDFUL APPROACH

Intermittent fasting is often introduced as a method to lose weight, manage blood sugar levels, or boost energy. But it can be more. For many, it becomes a powerful shift in how they relate to food, time, and themselves. It is not just about skipping meals or adjusting eating windows.

It is about creating space. Physically, mentally, and spiritually.

In a world where we are constantly consuming information, noise, and calories, fasting offers something rare: a pause. That pause can reveal patterns, challenge habits, and open a quiet path back to awareness.

And in that awareness, something begins to reset. You notice your hunger more clearly. You listen to your body. You start to choose instead of react. That is where growth begins.

This journal is not a rulebook. It is a companion. It offers structure, yes, but also provides opportunities for reflection. You will be invited to observe your progress, your feelings, and your choices without judgment.

To slow down and ask more profound questions. Why am I eating now? What am I truly hungry for?

Fasting can become a mindful act and even a spiritual one. It has long been a tool for self-discipline, clarity, and alignment across many traditions. Whether you walk a formal spiritual path or simply wish to live with more intention, fasting can support that journey.

When practiced with care, it becomes more than just a tool for health. It becomes a daily moment of integrity.

This is your reset. A chance to reconnect with simplicity. To develop a more respectful relationship with food. To replace urgency with presence. To shift from seeking more to appreciating enough.

You are not being asked to be perfect. You are simply being invited to show up. To be curious. To be kind to yourself. And to begin again, one moment at a time.

"You have power over your mind, not outside events.
Realize this, and you will find strength."
- Marcus Aurelius

Let this journal be a place of intention.
A place of small steps and steady shifts.
A place where change begins gently but surely from the inside out.

12 WEEKS
OF FASTING TRACKING

YOUR JOURNEY
STARTS HERE

Remember to use your weight tracker.
Download your Excel file from the hub.

WEEK 1 - DAY 1 DATE:

What kind of fast are you doing?

If your fast is longer than one day, what day are you on?

How well did you sleep last night?

What exercise have you done today?

What were your energy levels like throughout the day?

Daily Reflection

- What went well today and what would you change?
- Describe your emotions during your fast.
- How did you feel after completing your fast?

Did you drink enough water today?

WEEK 1 - DAY 2 DATE:

What kind of fast are you doing?

If your fast is longer than one day, what day are you on?

How well did you sleep last night?

What exercise have you done today?

What were your energy levels like throughout the day?

Daily Reflection

- What went well today and what would you change?
- Describe your emotions during your fast.
- How did you feel after completing your fast?

Did you drink enough water today?

WEEK 1 - DAY 3 DATE:

What kind of fast are you doing?

If your fast is longer than one day, what day are you on?

How well did you sleep last night?

What exercise have you done today?

What were your energy levels like throughout the day?

Daily Reflection

- What went well today and what would you change?
- Describe your emotions during your fast.
- How did you feel after completing your fast?

Did you drink enough water today?

WEEK 1 - DAY 4 DATE:

What kind of fast are you doing?

If your fast is longer than one day, what day are you on?

How well did you sleep last night?

What exercise have you done today?

What were your energy levels like throughout the day?

Daily Reflection

- What went well today and what would you change?
- Describe your emotions during your fast.
- How did you feel after completing your fast?

Did you drink enough water today?

WEEK 1 - DAY 5 DATE:

What kind of fast are you doing?

If your fast is longer than one day, what day are you on?

How well did you sleep last night?

What exercise have you done today?

What were your energy levels like throughout the day?

Daily Reflection

- What went well today and what would you change?
- Describe your emotions during your fast.
- How did you feel after completing your fast?

Did you drink enough water today?

WEEK 1 - DAY 6 DATE:

What kind of fast are you doing?

If your fast is longer than one cay, what day are you on?

How well did you sleep last night?

What exercise have you done today?

What were your energy levels like throughout the day?

Daily Reflection

- What went well today and what would you change?
- Describe your emotions during your fast.
- How did you feel after completing your fast?

Did you drink enough water today?

WEEK 1 - DAY 7 DATE:

What kind of fast are you doing?

If your fast is longer than one day, what day are you on?

How well did you sleep last night?

What exercise have you done today?

What were your energy levels like throughout the day?

Daily Reflection

- What went well today and what would you change?
- Describe your emotions during your fast.
- How did you feel after completing your fast?

Did you drink enough water today?

THE WEEK THAT WAS

What was your weight at the end of this week?

What were your core body measurements?

Chest

Waist

Hips

Take a moment to reflect on the week—your wins, challenges, and insights. How did fasting feel, physically and emotionally? Did you notice any changes, surprises, or moments of growth? What would you tell your future self about this journey?

THE WEEK AHEAD

What are your sleeping goals?

What are your fasting goals?

What are your hydration goals?

What are your food goals?

What are your exercise goals?

"Every journey begins with a single choice."

Starting is the hardest part, but consistency turns effort into transformation. Trust the process, track your progress, and let small wins fuel your motivation.

WEEK 2 - DAY 1 DATE:

What kind of fast are you doing?

If your fast is longer than one day, what day are you on?

How well did you sleep last night?

What exercise have you done today?

What were your energy levels like throughout the day?

Daily Reflection

- What went well today and what would you change?
- Describe your emotions during your fast.
- How did you feel after completing your fast?

Did you drink enough water today?

WEEK 2 - DAY 2 DATE:

What kind of fast are you doing?

If your fast is longer than one day, what day are you on?

How well did you sleep last night?

What exercise have you done today?

What were your energy levels like throughout the day?

Daily Reflection

- What went well today and what would you change?
- Describe your emotions during your fast.
- How did you feel after completing your fast?

Did you drink enough water today?

WEEK 2 - DAY 3 DATE:

What kind of fast are you doing?

If your fast is longer than one day, what day are you on?

How well did you sleep last night?

What exercise have you done today?

What were your energy levels like throughout the day?

Daily Reflection

- What went well today and what would you change?
- Describe your emotions during your fast.
- How did you feel after completing your fast?

Did you drink enough water today?

WEEK 2 - DAY 4 DATE:

What kind of fast are you doing?

If your fast is longer than one day, what day are you on?

How well did you sleep last night?

What exercise have you done today?

What were your energy levels like throughout the day?

Daily Reflection

- What went well today and what would you change?
- Describe your emotions during your fast.
- How did you feel after completing your fast?

Did you drink enough water today?

WEEK 2 - DAY 5 DATE:

What kind of fast are you doing?

If your fast is longer than one day, what day are you on?

How well did you sleep last night?

What exercise have you done today?

What were your energy levels like throughout the day?

Daily Reflection

- What went well today and what would you change?
- Describe your emotions during your fast.
- How did you feel after completing your fast?

Did you drink enough water today?

WEEK 2 - DAY 6 DATE:

What kind of fast are you doing?

If your fast is longer than one day, what day are you on?

How well did you sleep last night?

What exercise have you done today?

What were your energy levels like throughout the day?

Daily Reflection

- What went well today and what would you change?
- Describe your emotions during your fast.
- How did you feel after completing your fast?

Did you drink enough water today?

WEEK 2 - DAY 7 DATE:

What kind of fast are you doing?

If your fast is longer than one day, what day are you on?

How well did you sleep last night?

What exercise have you done today?

What were your energy levels like throughout the day?

Daily Reflection

- What went well today and what would you change?
- Describe your emotions during your fast.
- How did you feel after completing your fast?

Did you drink enough water today?

THE WEEK THAT WAS

What was your weight at the end of this week?

What were your core body measurements?

Chest

Waist

Hips

Take a moment to reflect on the week—your wins, challenges, and insights. How did fasting feel, physically and emotionally? Did you notice any changes, surprises, or moments of growth? What would you tell your future self about this journey?

THE WEEK AHEAD

What are your sleeping goals?

What are your fasting goals?

What are your hydration goals?

What are your food goals?

What are your exercise goals?

"Fasting isn't about deprivation; it's about renewal."

Each fast gives your body the space to reset and heal. Instead of focusing on what you're skipping, celebrate what you're gaining; strength, clarity, and control.

WEEK 3 - DAY 1 DATE:

What kind of fast are you doing?

If your fast is longer than one day, what day are you on?

How well did you sleep last night?

What exercise have you done today?

What were your energy levels like throughout the day?

Daily Reflection

- What went well today and what would you change?
- Describe your emotions during your fast.
- How did you feel after completing your fast?

Did you drink enough water today?

WEEK 3 - DAY 2 DATE:

What kind of fast are you doing?

If your fast is longer than one day, what day are you on?

How well did you sleep last night?

What exercise have you done today?

What were your energy levels like throughout the day?

Daily Reflection

- What went well today and what would you change?
- Describe your emotions during your fast.
- How did you feel after completing your fast?

Did you drink enough water today?

WEEK 3 - DAY 3 DATE:

What kind of fast are you doing?

If your fast is longer than one day, what day are you on?

How well did you sleep last night?

What exercise have you done today?

What were your energy levels like throughout the day?

Daily Reflection

- What went well today and what would you change?
- Describe your emotions during your fast.
- How did you feel after completing your fast?

Did you drink enough water today?

WEEK 3 - DAY 4 DATE:

What kind of fast are you doing?

If your fast is longer than one day, what day are you on?

How well did you sleep last night?

What exercise have you done today?

What were your energy levels like throughout the cay?

Daily Reflection

- What went well today and what would you change?
- Describe your emotions during your fast.
- How did you feel after completing your fast?

Did you drink enough water today?

WEEK 3 - DAY 5 DATE:

What kind of fast are you doing?

If your fast is longer than one day, what day are you on?

How well did you sleep last night?

What exercise have you done today?

What were your energy levels like throughout the day?

Daily Reflection

- What went well today and what would you change?
- Describe your emotions during your fast.
- How did you feel after completing your fast?

Did you drink enough water today?

WEEK 3 - DAY 6 DATE:

What kind of fast are you doing?

If your fast is longer than one day, what day are you on?

How well did you sleep last night?

What exercise have you done today?

What were your energy levels like throughout the day?

Daily Reflection

- What went well today and what would you change?
- Describe your emotions during your fast.
- How did you feel after completing your fast?

Did you drink enough water today?

WEEK 3 - DAY 7 DATE:

What kind of fast are you doing?

If your fast is longer than one day, what day are you on?

How well did you sleep last night?

What exercise have you done today?

What were your energy levels like throughout the day?

Daily Reflection

- What went well today and what would you change?
- Describe your emotions during your fast.
- How did you feel after completing your fast?

Did you drink enough water today?

THE WEEK THAT WAS

What was your weight at the end of this week?

What were your core body measurements?

Chest

Waist

Hips

Take a moment to reflect on the week—your wins, challenges, and insights. How did fasting feel, physically and emotionally? Did you notice any changes, surprises, or moments of growth? What would you tell your future self about this journey?

THE WEEK AHEAD

What are your sleeping goals?

What are your fasting goals?

What are your hydration goals?

What are your food goals?

What are your exercise goals?

"Discipline is just choosing what you want most over what you want now."

Hunger is temporary, but the rewards of patience and persistence are lasting. Stay focused, and remember why you started.

WEEK 4 - DAY 1 DATE:

What kind of fast are you doing?

If your fast is longer than one day, what day are you on?

How well did you sleep last night?

What exercise have you done today?

What were your energy levels like throughout the day?

Daily Reflection

- What went well today and what would you change?
- Describe your emotions during your fast.
- How did you feel after completing your fast?

Did you drink enough water today?

WEEK 4 - DAY 2 DATE:

What kind of fast are you doing?

If your fast is longer than one day, what day are you on?

How well did you sleep last night?

What exercise have you done today?

What were your energy levels like throughout the day?

Daily Reflection

- What went well today and what would you change?
- Describe your emotions during your fast.
- How did you feel after completing your fast?

Did you drink enough water today?

WEEK 4 - DAY 3 DATE:

What kind of fast are you doing?

If your fast is longer than one day, what day are you on?

How well did you sleep last night?

What exercise have you done today?

What were your energy levels like throughout the day?

Daily Reflection

- What went well today and what would you change?
- Describe your emotions during your fast.
- How did you feel after completing your fast?

Did you drink enough water today?

WEEK 4 - DAY 4 DATE:

What kind of fast are you doing?

If your fast is longer than one day, what day are you on?

How well did you sleep last night?

What exercise have you done today?

What were your energy levels like throughout the day?

Daily Reflection

- What went well today and what would you change?
- Describe your emotions during your fast.
- How did you feel after completing your fast?

Did you drink enough water today?

WEEK 4 - DAY 5 DATE:

What kind of fast are you doing?

If your fast is longer than one day, what day are you on?

How well did you sleep last night?

What exercise have you done today?

What were your energy levels like throughout the day?

Daily Reflection

- What went well today and what would you change?
- Describe your emotions during your fast.
- How did you feel after completing your fast?

Did you drink enough water today?

WEEK 4 - DAY 6 DATE:

What kind of fast are you doing?

If your fast is longer than one day, what day are you on?

How well did you sleep last night?

What exercise have you done today?

What were your energy levels like throughout the day?

Daily Reflection

- What went well today and what would you change?
- Describe your emotions during your fast.
- How did you feel after completing your fast?

Did you drink enough water today?

WEEK 4 - DAY 7 DATE:

What kind of fast are you doing?

If your fast is longer than one day, what day are you on?

How well did you sleep last night?

What exercise have you done today?

What were your energy levels like throughout the day?

Daily Reflection

- What went well today and what would you change?
- Describe your emotions during your fast.
- How did you feel after completing your fast?

Did you drink enough water today?

THE WEEK THAT WAS

What was your weight at the end of this week?

What were your core body measurements?

Chest

Waist

Hips

Take a moment to reflect on the week—your wins, challenges, and insights. How did fasting feel, physically and emotionally? Did you notice any changes, surprises, or moments of growth? What would you tell your future self about this journey?

THE WEEK AHEAD

What are your sleeping goals?

What are your fasting goals?

What are your hydration goals?

What are your food goals?

What are your exercise goals?

"Your body hears everything your mind says."

Speak kindly to yourself. A missed fast or an imperfect meal doesn't erase progress; what matters is how you move forward.

WEEK 5 - DAY 1 DATE:

What kind of fast are you doing?

If your fast is longer than one day, what day are you on?

How well did you sleep last night?

What exercise have you done today?

What were your energy levels like throughout the day?

Daily Reflection

- What went well today and what would you change?
- Describe your emotions during your fast.
- How did you feel after completing your fast?

Did you drink enough water today?

WEEK 5 - DAY 2 DATE:

What kind of fast are you doing?

If your fast is longer than one day, what day are you on?

How well did you sleep last night?

What exercise have you done today?

What were your energy levels like throughout the day?

Daily Reflection

- What went well today and what would you change?
- Describe your emotions during your fast.
- How did you feel after completing your fast?

Did you drink enough water today?

WEEK 5 - DAY 3 DATE:

What kind of fast are you doing?

If your fast is longer than one day, what day are you on?

How well did you sleep last night?

What exercise have you done today?

What were your energy levels like throughout the day?

Daily Reflection

- What went well today and what would you change?
- Describe your emotions during your fast.
- How did you feel after completing your fast?

Did you drink enough water today?

WEEK 5 - DAY 4 DATE:

What kind of fast are you doing?

If your fast is longer than one day, what day are you on?

How well did you sleep last night?

What exercise have you done today?

What were your energy levels like throughout the day?

Daily Reflection

- What went well today and what would you change?
- Describe your emotions during your fast.
- How did you feel after completing your fast?

Did you drink enough water today?

WEEK 5 - DAY 5 DATE:

What kind of fast are you doing?

If your fast is longer than one day, what day are you on?

How well did you sleep last night?

What exercise have you done today?

What were your energy levels like throughout the day?

Daily Reflection

- What went well today and what would you change?
- Describe your emotions during your fast.
- How did you feel after completing your fast?

Did you drink enough water today?

WEEK 5 - DAY 6 DATE:

What kind of fast are you doing?

If your fast is longer than one day, what day are you on?

How well did you sleep last night?

What exercise have you done today?

What were your energy levels like throughout the day?

Daily Reflection

- What went well today and what would you change?
- Describe your emotions during your fast.
- How did you feel after completing your fast?

Did you drink enough water today?

WEEK 5 - DAY 7 DATE:

What kind of fast are you doing?

If your fast is longer than one day, what day are you on?

How well did you sleep last night?

What exercise have you done today?

What were your energy levels like throughout the day?

Daily Reflection

- What went well today and what would you change?
- Describe your emotions during your fast.
- How did you feel after completing your fast?

Did you drink enough water today?

THE WEEK THAT WAS

What was your weight at the end of this week?

What were your core body measurements?

Chest

Waist

Hips

Take a moment to reflect on the week—your wins, challenges, and insights. How did fasting feel, physically and emotionally? Did you notice any changes, surprises, or moments of growth? What would you tell your future self about this journey?

THE WEEK AHEAD

What are your sleeping goals?

What are your fasting goals?

What are your hydration goals?

What are your food goals?

What are your exercise goals?

"Progress isn't always visible, but it's always happening."

Some changes are felt before they're seen. Trust that your body is adapting, even on the weeks the scale doesn't move.

WEEK 6 - DAY 1 DATE:

What kind of fast are you doing?

If your fast is longer than one day, what day are you on?

How well did you sleep last night?

What exercise have you done today?

What were your energy levels like throughout the day?

Daily Reflection

- What went well today and what would you change?
- Describe your emotions during your fast.
- How did you feel after completing your fast?

Did you drink enough water today?

WEEK 6 - DAY 2 DATE:

What kind of fast are you doing?

If your fast is longer than one day, what day are you on?

How well did you sleep last night?

What exercise have you done today?

What were your energy levels like throughout the day?

Daily Reflection

- What went well today and what would you change?
- Describe your emotions during your fast.
- How did you feel after completing your fast?

Did you drink enough water today?

WEEK 6 - DAY 3 DATE:

What kind of fast are you doing?

If your fast is longer than one day, what day are you on?

How well did you sleep last night?

What exercise have you done today?

What were your energy levels like throughout the day?

Daily Reflection

- What went well today and what would you change?
- Describe your emotions during your fast.
- How did you feel after completing your fast?

Did you drink enough water today?

WEEK 6 - DAY 4 DATE:

What kind of fast are you doing?

If your fast is longer than one day, what day are you on?

How well did you sleep last night?

What exercise have you done today?

What were your energy levels like throughout the day?

Daily Reflection

- What went well today and what would you change?
- Describe your emotions during your fast.
- How did you feel after completing your fast?

Did you drink enough water today?

WEEK 6 - DAY 5 DATE:

What kind of fast are you doing?

If your fast is longer than one day, what day are you on?

How well did you sleep last night?

What exercise have you done today?

What were your energy levels like throughout the day?

Daily Reflection

- What went well today and what would you change?
- Describe your emotions during your fast.
- How did you feel after completing your fast?

Did you drink enough water today?

WEEK 6 - DAY 6 DATE:

What kind of fast are you doing?

If your fast is longer than one day, what day are you on?

How well did you sleep last night?

What exercise have you done today?

What were your energy levels like throughout the day?

Daily Reflection

- What went well today and what would you change?
- Describe your emotions during your fast.
- How did you feel after completing your fast?

Did you drink enough water today?

WEEK 6 - DAY 7 DATE:

What kind of fast are you doing?

If your fast is longer than one day, what day are you on?

How well did you sleep last night?

What exercise have you done today?

What were your energy levels like throughout the day?

Daily Reflection

- What went well today and what would you change?
- Describe your emotions during your fast.
- How did you feel after completing your fast?

Did you drink enough water today?

THE WEEK THAT WAS

What was your weight at the end of this week?

What were your core body measurements?

Chest

Waist

Hips

Take a moment to reflect on the week—your wins, challenges, and insights. How did fasting feel, physically and emotionally? Did you notice any changes, surprises, or moments of growth? What would you tell your future self about this journey?

THE WEEK AHEAD

What are your sleeping goals?

What are your fasting goals?

What are your hydration goals?

What are your food goals?

What are your exercise goals?

"You are not starting over; you are starting from experience."

Every challenge teaches you something new. Use what you've learned, adjust your plan if needed, and keep going.

WEEK 7 - DAY 1 DATE:

What kind of fast are you doing?

If your fast is longer than one day, what day are you on?

How well did you sleep last night?

What exercise have you done today?

What were your energy levels like throughout the day?

Daily Reflection

- What went well today and what would you change?
- Describe your emotions during your fast.
- How did you feel after completing your fast?

Did you drink enough water today?

WEEK 7 - DAY 2 DATE:

What kind of fast are you doing?

If your fast is longer than one day, what day are you on?

How well did you sleep last night?

What exercise have you done today?

What were your energy levels like throughout the day?

Daily Reflection

- What went well today and what would you change?
- Describe your emotions during your fast.
- How did you feel after completing your fast?

Did you drink enough water today?

WEEK 7 - DAY 3 DATE:

What kind of fast are you doing?

If your fast is longer than one day, what day are you on?

How well did you sleep last night?

What exercise have you done today?

What were your energy levels like throughout the day?

Daily Reflection

- What went well today and what would you change?
- Describe your emotions during your fast.
- How did you feel after completing your fast?

Did you drink enough water today?

WEEK 7 - DAY 4 DATE:

What kind of fast are you doing?

If your fast is longer than one day, what day are you on?

How well did you sleep last night?

What exercise have you done today?

What were your energy levels like throughout the day?

Daily Reflection

- What went well today and what would you change?
- Describe your emotions during your fast.
- How did you feel after completing your fast?

Did you drink enough water today?

WEEK 7 - DAY 5 DATE:

What kind of fast are you doing?

If your fast is longer than one day, what day are you on?

How well did you sleep last night?

What exercise have you done today?

What were your energy levels like throughout the day?

Daily Reflection

- What went well today and what would you change?
- Describe your emotions during your fast.
- How did you feel after completing your fast?

Did you drink enough water today?

WEEK 7 - DAY 6 DATE:

What kind of fast are you doing?

If your fast is longer than one day, what day are you on?

How well did you sleep last night?

What exercise have you done today?

What were your energy levels like throughout the day?

Daily Reflection

- What went well today and what would you change?
- Describe your emotions during your fast.
- How did you feel after completing your fast?

Did you drink enough water today?

WEEK 7 - DAY 7 DATE:

What kind of fast are you doing?

If your fast is longer than one day, what day are you on?

How well did you sleep last night?

What exercise have you done today?

What were your energy levels like throughout the day?

Daily Reflection

- What went well today and what would you change?
- Describe your emotions during your fast.
- How did you feel after completing your fast?

Did you drink enough water today?

THE WEEK THAT WAS

What was your weight at the end of this week?

What were your core body measurements?

Chest

Waist

Hips

Take a moment to reflect on the week—your wins, challenges, and insights. How did fasting feel, physically and emotionally? Did you notice any changes, surprises, or moments of growth? What would you tell your future self about this journey?

THE WEEK AHEAD

What are your sleeping goals?

What are your fasting goals?

What are your hydration goals?

What are your food goals?

What are your exercise goals?

"Success is built on small, daily choices."

It's not about being perfect; it's about being persistent. One mindful decision at a time will lead to lasting change.

WEEK 8 - DAY 1 DATE:

What kind of fast are you doing?

If your fast is longer than one day, what day are you on?

How well did you sleep last night?

What exercise have you done today?

What were your energy levels like throughout the day?

Daily Reflection

- What went well today and what would you change?
- Describe your emotions during your fast.
- How did you feel after completing your fast?

Did you drink enough water today?

WEEK 8 - DAY 2 DATE:

What kind of fast are you doing?

If your fast is longer than one day, what day are you on?

How well did you sleep last night?

What exercise have you done today?

What were your energy levels like throughout the day?

Daily Reflection

- What went well today and what would you change?
- Describe your emotions during your fast.
- How did you feel after completing your fast?

Did you drink enough water today?

WEEK 8 - DAY 3 DATE:

What kind of fast are you doing?

If your fast is longer than one day, what day are you on?

How well did you sleep last night?

What exercise have you done today?

What were your energy levels like throughout the day?

Daily Reflection

- What went well today and what would you change?
- Describe your emotions during your fast.
- How did you feel after completing your fast?

Did you drink enough water today?

WEEK 8 - DAY 4 DATE:

What kind of fast are you doing?

If your fast is longer than one day, what day are you on?

How well did you sleep last night?

What exercise have you done today?

What were your energy levels like throughout the day?

Daily Reflection

- What went well today and what would you change?
- Describe your emotions during your fast.
- How did you feel after completing your fast?

Did you drink enough water today?

WEEK 8 - DAY 5 DATE:

What kind of fast are you doing?

If your fast is longer than one day, what day are you on?

How well did you sleep last night?

What exercise have you done today?

What were your energy levels like throughout the day?

Daily Reflection

- What went well today and what would you change?
- Describe your emotions during your fast.
- How did you feel after completing your fast?

Did you drink enough water today?

WEEK 8 - DAY 6 DATE:

What kind of fast are you doing?

If your fast is longer than one day, what day are you on?

How well did you sleep last night?

What exercise have you done today?

What were your energy levels like throughout the day?

Daily Reflection

- What went well today and what would you change?
- Describe your emotions during your fast.
- How did you feel after completing your fast?

Did you drink enough water today?

WEEK 8 - DAY 7 DATE:

What kind of fast are you doing?

If your fast is longer than one day, what day are you on?

How well did you sleep last night?

What exercise have you done today?

What were your energy levels like throughout the day?

Daily Reflection

- What went well today and what would you change?
- Describe your emotions during your fast.
- How did you feel after completing your fast?

Did you drink enough water today?

THE WEEK THAT WAS

What was your weight at the end of this week?

What were your core body measurements?

Chest

Waist

Hips

Take a moment to reflect on the week—your wins, challenges, and insights. How did fasting feel, physically and emotionally? Did you notice any changes, surprises, or moments of growth? What would you tell your future self about this journey?

THE WEEK AHEAD

What are your sleeping goals?

What are your fasting goals?

What are your hydration goals?

What are your food goals?

What are your exercise goals?

"Your habits shape your future."

Fasting is more than an eating pattern; it's a mindset, a lifestyle. The discipline you build here will empower other areas of your life.

WEEK 9 - DAY 1 DATE:

What kind of fast are you doing?

If your fast is longer than one day, what day are you on?

How well did you sleep last night?

What exercise have you done today?

What were your energy levels like throughout the day?

Daily Reflection

- What went well today and what would you change?
- Describe your emotions during your fast.
- How did you feel after completing your fast?

Did you drink enough water today?

WEEK 9 - DAY 2 DATE:

What kind of fast are you doing?

If your fast is longer than one day, what day are you on?

How well did you sleep last night?

What exercise have you done today?

What were your energy levels like throughout the day?

Daily Reflection

- What went well today and what would you change?
- Describe your emotions during your fast.
- How did you feel after completing your fast?

Did you drink enough water today?

WEEK 9 - DAY 3 DATE:

What kind of fast are you doing?

If your fast is longer than one day, what day are you on?

How well did you sleep last night?

What exercise have you done today?

What were your energy levels like throughout the day?

Daily Reflection

- What went well today and what would you change?
- Describe your emotions during your fast.
- How did you feel after completing your fast?

Did you drink enough water today?

WEEK 9 - DAY 4 DATE:

What kind of fast are you doing?

If your fast is longer than one day, what day are you on?

How well did you sleep last night?

What exercise have you done today?

What were your energy levels like throughout the day?

Daily Reflection

- What went well today and what would you change?
- Describe your emotions during your fast.
- How did you feel after completing your fast?

Did you drink enough water today?

WEEK 9 - DAY 5 DATE:

What kind of fast are you doing?

If your fast is longer than one day, what day are you on?

How well did you sleep last night?

What exercise have you done today?

What were your energy levels like throughout the day?

Daily Reflection

- What went well today and what would you change?
- Describe your emotions during your fast.
- How did you feel after completing your fast?

Did you drink enough water today?

WEEK 9 - DAY 6 DATE:

What kind of fast are you doing?

If your fast is longer than one day, what day are you on?

How well did you sleep last night?

What exercise have you done today?

What were your energy levels like throughout the day?

Daily Reflection

- What went well today and what would you change?
- Describe your emotions during your fast.
- How did you feel after completing your fast?

Did you drink enough water today?

WEEK 9 - DAY 7 DATE:

What kind of fast are you doing?

If your fast is longer than one day, what day are you on?

How well did you sleep last night?

What exercise have you done today?

What were your energy levels like throughout the day?

Daily Reflection

- What went well today and what would you change?
- Describe your emotions during your fast.
- How did you feel after completing your fast?

Did you drink enough water today?

THE WEEK THAT WAS

What was your weight at the end of this week?

What were your core body measurements?

Chest

Waist

Hips

Take a moment to reflect on the week—your wins, challenges, and insights. How did fasting feel, physically and emotionally? Did you notice any changes, surprises, or moments of growth? What would you tell your future self about this journey?

THE WEEK AHEAD

What are your sleeping goals?

What are your fasting goals?

What are your hydration goals?

What are your food goals?

What are your exercise goals?

"Energy flows where attention goes."

Instead of obsessing over numbers, focus on how you feel; lighter, stronger, more in control. The results will follow.

WEEK 10 - DAY 1 DATE:

What kind of fast are you doing?

If your fast is longer than one day, what day are you on?

How well did you sleep last night?

What exercise have you done today?

What were your energy levels like throughout the day?

Daily Reflection

- What went well today and what would you change?
- Describe your emotions during your fast.
- How did you feel after completing your fast?

Did you drink enough water today?

WEEK 10 - DAY 2 DATE:

What kind of fast are you doing?

If your fast is longer than one day, what day are you on?

How well did you sleep last night?

What exercise have you done today?

What were your energy levels like throughout the day?

Daily Reflection

- What went well today and what would you change?
- Describe your emotions during your fast.
- How did you feel after completing your fast?

Did you drink enough water today?

WEEK 10 - DAY 3 DATE:

What kind of fast are you doing?

If your fast is longer than one day, what day are you on?

How well did you sleep last night?

What exercise have you done today?

What were your energy levels like throughout the day?

Daily Reflection

- What went well today and what would you change?
- Describe your emotions during your fast.
- How did you feel after completing your fast?

Did you drink enough water today?

WEEK 10 - DAY 4 DATE:

What kind of fast are you doing?

If your fast is longer than one day, what day are you on?

How well did you sleep last night?

What exercise have you done today?

What were your energy levels like throughout the day?

Daily Reflection

- What went well today and what would you change?
- Describe your emotions during your fast.
- How did you feel after completing your fast?

Did you drink enough water today?

WEEK 10 - DAY 5 DATE:

What kind of fast are you doing?

If your fast is longer than one day, what day are you on?

How well did you sleep last night?

What exercise have you done today?

What were your energy levels like throughout the day?

Daily Reflection

- What went well today and what would you change?
- Describe your emotions during your fast.
- How did you feel after completing your fast?

Did you drink enough water today?

WEEK 10 - DAY 6 DATE:

What kind of fast are you doing?

If your fast is longer than one day, what day are you on?

How well did you sleep last night?

What exercise have you done today?

What were your energy levels like throughout the day?

Daily Reflection

- What went well today and what would you change?
- Describe your emotions during your fast.
- How did you feel after completing your fast?

Did you drink enough water today?

WEEK 10 - DAY 7 DATE:

What kind of fast are you doing?

If your fast is longer than one day, what day are you on?

How well did you sleep last night?

What exercise have you done today?

What were your energy levels like throughout the day?

Daily Reflection

- What went well today and what would you change?
- Describe your emotions during your fast.
- How did you feel after completing your fast?

Did you drink enough water today?

THE WEEK THAT WAS

What was your weight at the end of this week?

What were your core body measurements?

Chest

Waist

Hips

Take a moment to reflect on the week—your wins, challenges, and insights. How did fasting feel, physically and emotionally? Did you notice any changes, surprises, or moments of growth? What would you tell your future self about this journey?

THE WEEK AHEAD

What are your sleeping goals?

What are your fasting goals?

What are your hydration goals?

What are your food goals?

What are your exercise goals?

"The way you do one thing is the way you do everything."

How you commit to this journey reflects your approach to life. Show up for yourself with intention and purpose.

WEEK 11 - DAY 1 DATE:

What kind of fast are you doing?

If your fast is longer than one day, what day are you on?

How well did you sleep last night?

What exercise have you done today?

What were your energy levels like throughout the day?

Daily Reflection

- What went well today and what would you change?
- Describe your emotions during your fast.
- How did you feel after completing your fast?

Did you drink enough water today?

WEEK 11 - DAY 2 DATE:

What kind of fast are you doing?

If your fast is longer than one day, what day are you on?

How well did you sleep last night?

What exercise have you done today?

What were your energy levels like throughout the day?

Daily Reflection

- What went well today and what would you change?
- Describe your emotions during your fast.
- How did you feel after completing your fast?

Did you drink enough water today?

WEEK 11 - DAY 3 DATE:

What kind of fast are you doing?

If your fast is longer than one day, what day are you on?

How well did you sleep last night?

What exercise have you done today?

What were your energy levels like throughout the day?

Daily Reflection

- What went well today and what would you change?
- Describe your emotions during your fast.
- How did you feel after completing your fast?

Did you drink enough water today?

WEEK 11 - DAY 4 DATE:

What kind of fast are you doing?

If your fast is longer than one day, what day are you on?

How well did you sleep last night?

What exercise have you done today?

What were your energy levels like throughout the day?

Daily Reflection

- What went well today and what would you change?
- Describe your emotions during your fast.
- How did you feel after completing your fast?

Did you drink enough water today?

WEEK 11 - DAY 5 DATE:

What kind of fast are you doing?

If your fast is longer than one day, what day are you on?

How well did you sleep last night?

What exercise have you done today?

What were your energy levels like throughout the day?

Daily Reflection

- What went well today and what would you change?
- Describe your emotions during your fast.
- How did you feel after completing your fast?

Did you drink enough water today?

WEEK 11 - DAY 6 DATE:

What kind of fast are you doing?

If your fast is longer than one day, what day are you on?

How well did you sleep last night?

What exercise have you done today?

What were your energy levels like throughout the day?

Daily Reflection

- What went well today and what would you change?
- Describe your emotions during your fast.
- How did you feel after completing your fast?

Did you drink enough water today?

WEEK 11 - DAY 7 DATE:

What kind of fast are you doing?

If your fast is longer than one day, what day are you on?

How well did you sleep last night?

What exercise have you done today?

What were your energy levels like throughout the day?

Daily Reflection

- What went well today and what would you change?
- Describe your emotions during your fast.
- How did you feel after completing your fast?

Did you drink enough water today?

THE WEEK THAT WAS

What was your weight at the end of this week?

What were your core body measurements?

Chest

Waist

Hips

Take a moment to reflect on the week—your wins, challenges, and insights. How did fasting feel, physically and emotionally? Did you notice any changes, surprises, or moments of growth? What would you tell your future self about this journey?

THE WEEK AHEAD

What are your sleeping goals?

What are your fasting goals?

What are your hydration goals?

What are your food goals?

What are your exercise goals?

"You don't have to do it fast; you just have to do it."

Change takes time, and progress looks different for everyone. Honor your own pace, and trust that you're getting stronger every day.

WEEK 12 - DAY 1 DATE:

What kind of fast are you doing?

If your fast is longer than one day, what day are you on?

How well did you sleep last night?

What exercise have you done today?

What were your energy levels like throughout the day?

Daily Reflection

- What went well today and what would you change?
- Describe your emotions during your fast.
- How did you feel after completing your fast?

Did you drink enough water today?

WEEK 12 - DAY 2 DATE:

What kind of fast are you doing?

If your fast is longer than one day, what day are you on?

How well did you sleep last night?

What exercise have you done today?

What were your energy levels like throughout the day?

Daily Reflection

- What went well today and what would you change?
- Describe your emotions during your fast.
- How did you feel after completing your fast?

Did you drink enough water today?

WEEK 12 - DAY 3 DATE:

What kind of fast are you doing?

If your fast is longer than one day, what day are you on?

How well did you sleep last night?

What exercise have you done today?

What were your energy levels like throughout the day?

Daily Reflection

- What went well today and what would you change?
- Describe your emotions during your fast.
- How did you feel after completing your fast?

Did you drink enough water today?

WEEK 12 - DAY 4 DATE:

What kind of fast are you doing?

If your fast is longer than one day, what day are you on?

How well did you sleep last night?

What exercise have you done today?

What were your energy levels like throughout the day?

Daily Reflection

- What went well today and what would you change?
- Describe your emotions during your fast.
- How did you feel after completing your fast?

Did you drink enough water today?

WEEK 12 - DAY 5 DATE:

What kind of fast are you doing?

If your fast is longer than one day, what day are you on?

How well did you sleep last night?

What exercise have you done today?

What were your energy levels like throughout the day?

Daily Reflection

- What went well today and what would you change?
- Describe your emotions during your fast.
- How did you feel after completing your fast?

Did you drink enough water today?

WEEK 12 - DAY 6 DATE:

What kind of fast are you doing?

If your fast is longer than one day, what day are you on?

How well did you sleep last night?

What exercise have you done today?

What were your energy levels like throughout the day?

Daily Reflection

- What went well today and what would you change?
- Describe your emotions during your fast.
- How did you feel after completing your fast?

Did you drink enough water today?

WEEK 12 - DAY 7 DATE:

What kind of fast are you doing?

If your fast is longer than one day, what day are you on?

How well did you sleep last night?

What exercise have you done today?

What were your energy levels like throughout the day?

Daily Reflection

- What went well today and what would you change?
- Describe your emotions during your fast.
- How did you feel after completing your fast?

Did you drink enough water today?

THE WEEK THAT WAS

What was your weight at the end of this week?

What were your core body measurements?

Chest

Waist

Hips

Take a moment to reflect on the week—your wins, challenges, and insights. How did fasting feel, physically and emotionally? Did you notice any changes, surprises, or moments of growth? What would you tell your future self about this journey?

YOU MADE IT!

Take a deep breath and let that truth settle in. This wasn't just about food choices or sticking to a plan. It was about choosing yourself every day. About learning to listen to your body, respect its signals, and build a relationship of trust with your well-being.

This journal has become more than a record. It has held your reflections, small triumphs, and the deeper reasons that brought you here. You began this journey to feel better, to live with more energy, and to shape a life aligned with your intentions.

Before you close this chapter, take a moment to reflect using the following two pages.

Ask yourself:
- What have I discovered about myself?
- What am I most proud of?
- How do I feel differently now, in body, mind, and spirit?

Be proud

Be kind to yourself

Let your progress inspire you

When you're ready, consider starting your next 12-week chapter. Continuing with a second journal is not just about momentum; it's a statement of commitment to your long-term health and growth. That decision often brings clarity, confidence, and renewed energy.

If you order your next journal from the Impisi Media website, you will receive a 15% discount by using the code **website15** at checkout.

Here's to your next step, keep going, you're worth it.

REFLECTION ON YOUR JOURNEY

THANK YOU FOR READING

If you found this book helpful, I'd greatly appreciate it if you could take a moment to leave a review on Amazon. Your feedback not only helps me improve but also assists other readers in finding the right resources. Scan the QR code to share your thoughts.

SCAN ME

I appreciate your support!

ABOUT THE AUTHOR

Ellen Sedge is a seasoned entrepreneur whose career has evolved from mastering financial systems to mentoring others on their path to personal and professional growth. With a background spanning from simple bookkeeping to complex financial systems, she founded a training academy early in her career and later worked as an independent consultant for medium-sized businesses.

In search of better work-life balance, Ellen transitioned to running a home-based business, later launching and managing two more businesses abroad. Her extensive travel across five continents has enriched her perspective on life, resilience, and intentional living.

Ellen draws from her firsthand experience in time management, discipline, and lifestyle design; skills honed through decades of independent work. Her books, including *Mastering Time for Productivity*, *The Wolf's Edge*, and *Reset with Intermittent Fasting*, reflect her passion for empowering others to take control of their time, mindset, and well-being.

ABOUT THE PUBLISHER

ImpisiTM Media is a dynamic publishing company dedicated to creating and distributing high-quality intellectual property, including books, e-books, audiobooks, and journals.

Our content is crafted to inform, inspire, and empower a global audience. Our commitment to innovation and excellence drives us to deliver content that resonates and adds value to our readers and listeners.

Visit our website https://impisimedia.com

Follow Us on Social Media

@impisimedia

Made in the USA
Coppell, TX
23 November 2025

63775736R00085